Low Fodmap Diet

A Comprehensive Guide To Treating Irritable Bowel
Syndrome And Other Digestive Disorders

*(Low-fodmap And Delectable Recipes For Inflammatory
Bowel Disease Relief And Remission)*

Rajinder Crawford

TABLE OF CONTENT

Introduction

Do you have irritable bowel syndrome (IBS), Crohn's disease, ulserative colitis, or one of the numerous other forms of food intolerance? If this describes you, the low-FODMAP diet may be worth trying.

When it easy come to treating rats with chronic digestive health issues, physicians and dietitians recommend the Low FODMAP diet. The Low FODMAP diet is beneficial for the treatment of Irritable Bowel Syndrome (IBS) and other related conditions. The diet recommends avoiding several meals because of their poor digestibility. Following the diet can alleviate IBS symptoms in up to 80% of individuals.

Many people with digestive problems have discovered that certain substances affect their stomachs. In certain instances, it may just take considerable time and trial and error to determine which foods cause an allergic reaction. Studies have demonstrated that our bodies' digestive enzymes have difficulty assimilating certain types of carbohydrates, sugars, and dietary fibers.

In sontrat, the beneficial bacteria in our digestive system convert them into a substance that is safe for human consumption. It's unfortunate that avoiding these foods and consuming only low-FODMAP foods is the best way to alleviate the discomfort caused by certain foods.

A low-FODMAP diet may help those with digestive issues such as bloating, diarrhea, or irritable bowel syndrome (IBS).

Who should adhere to a FODMAP-restricted diet, and why? The low

FODMAP diet is also known as the FODMAP elimination diet. This diet, which is intended to be followed for a brief period, is low in dietary molecules known as FODMAPs.

In this sentence, 'it' refers to:

• Fermentable foods can be digested (fermented) by bacteria in the stomach.

• Oligosaccharides are short-chain carbohydrates; oligo refers to a small quantity. These molecules are composed of a multitude of carbohydrates.

• Two-sugar compounds are referred to as dassharde. This is a molecule composed of two sugars.

• The term "monoassharde" refers to the unique quality of this sugar. Only one sugar capsule is displayed here.

• And Poluol, which are essentially sugar-based alcoholic beverages (but won't get you inebriated!

Oligosaccharides, disaccharides, monosaccharides, and roluol are the four main saccharide groups that easy make up ur FODMAP. Each of these FODMAP categories has been assigned a unique moniker, and some of them may contain additional FODMAP categories.

• The oligosaccharide family is divided into two slae, frustan and galastan (or galasto-oligosaccharide or GOS for short). • Lastoe, a type of disaccharide, contains a single sugar moiety.

• Frustoe, also known as exse frustoe, is a form of monoassharde that contains only one sugar unit.

• Sorbitol and mannitol are two roluol derivatives.

For simplicity's sake, I will continue to refer to these molecules as FODMAPs. These are examples of short-chain sarbohudrates, which, if not adequately broken down, may promote fermentation in the large intestine (bowel). ntetnal dilatation and tretshng ossur result from the formation of carbon dioxide, hydrogen, and/or methane during fermentation.

The symptoms of soneuense include severe discomfort, stomach enlargement, and other symptoms of bloating and flatulence.

What does a limited FODMAP diet consist of? This regimen is commonly used to alleviate digestive issues, but it is also used to treat a variety of other conditions.

It may be advantageous for reron who have:

• Irritable Bowel Syndrome (IBS) • Other manifestations of Functional Gastrointestinal Disorder (FGID) • Bacterial proliferation in the small intestine (SIBO) • Certain auto-immune diseases and conditions, including (potentially) rheumatoid arthritis, multiple sclerosis, and eczema

• Certain foods may be responsible for your fibromyalgia or other health issues.

• Frequent migraines that must be treated with resuscitation food

• Crohn's disease, ulcerative colitis, and multiple sclerosis are all examples of inflammatory bowel disease (IBD).

Not to be confused with a diet's chemical intolerance, such as a low-hydantoin or low-salicylate diet.

What does a Low FODMAP diet entail? A low FODMAP diet restricts some carbohydrates, but it is not the same as a low-carb diet. It excludes high FODMAP foods and can be customized to exclude only those that trigger your symptoms. The acronym FODMAP stands for "Fermentable Oligosaccharides, Disaccharides, Monosaccharides, and Polyols."

The majority of individuals have no adverse reactions to FODMAPs; however, some individuals may experience bloating, gas, or diarrhea. Some individuals are sensitive to

FODMAPs because they absorb more fluid in the intestinal tract and produce more gas. They produce more alcohol because they ferment on the tongue more readily. The combination of additional fluid and increased gas may slow digestion, resulting in gas, bloating, diarrhea, or constipation.

Chapter 1: How To Adhere To The Low-Fodmap Diet

A low-FODMAP diet is more complex than you may believe and consists of three phases.

Stage 2 : Restristion

This stage involves avoiding all foods that are elevated in FODMAPs.

People who follow this diet often believe they should avoid all FODMAPs indefinitely, but this phase should only last between 6 and 8 weeks. This is because including FODMAPs in the diet is essential for digestive health.

Some patients experience symptom alleviation in the first week, while others require the full eight weeks. Once you have obtained sufficient alleviation from your digestive symptoms, you may proceed to the next stage.

Refer to the What If Your Symptoms Really do not Improve section if, after eight weeks, your gastrointestinal symptoms have not improved.

Stage 2: Reintrodustion

This stage involves reintroducing high-FODMAP foods systematically.

The significance of this is twofold:

• To determine which FODMAPs you can tolerate. Few individuals are receptive to all of them.

• Determine the quantity of FODMAPs that you can tolerate. This is referred to as our "threshold level."

In this term, you sample specified foods one by one over the course of three days each.

It is recommended that you embark on this journey with a trained dietitian who can guide you through the proper food choices.

It is important to note that you must maintain a low-FODMAP diet throughout this stage. Even if you can tolerate a specific high-FODMAP food, you must continue to reintroduce it until stage 6 .

It is also essential to remember that, unlike those with most food allergies, those with irritable bowel syndrome can tolerate small amounts of FODMAPs.

Latlu, despite the fact that digestive symptoms can be debilitating, they will not cause long-term harm to your body.

Stage 6 : Personalization

This is also referred to as the "modified low-FODMAP diet." In other words, you must still limit some FODMAPs. However, the quantity and temperature are tailored to your individual tolerance, as determined in Stage 2.

It is essential to reach this stage in order to enhance diet variety and flexibility. These characteristics are associated with enhanced long-term compliance, quality of life, and gastrointestinal health.

Chapter 2: Nutritional Deficiencies

Even if you are eating enough food, you may still be at risk for certain nutritional deficiencies if your diet is unbalanced. In addition, you may have nutritional deficiencies due to certain health or life conditions, such as pregnancy, or certain medications, such as high blood pressure medications. People who have had intestinal maladies or had a portion of their intestines surgically removed due to disease or obesity. also mau be at risk for vitamin defisiensies. Alcoholics are also at increased risk for nutritional deficiencies.

One of the most prevalent nutritional defenses is ron defensu anemia. Your blood requires iron in order to provide your body with oxygen; if you do not have enough iron, your blood will not function properly. Other nutritional deficiencies that can affect your blood count include deficiencies in vitamin B2 2, folate, and vitamin C.

Vtamn D deficiency may compromise the health of your bones, making it difficult for you to absorb and utilize sodium (another nutrient you may not be getting enough of). Although you can get vitamin D by going out in the sun, people who are concerned about skin cancer may end up with low vitamin D levels if they really do not get enough exposure.

Additional nutritional definitions include:

Berber: vitamin B2 deficiency (found in cereal husks).

Arboflavno: a low concentration of vitamin B2

Rellagra: low vitamin B6 levels

Rare: low levels of vitamin B10 cause a "pins and needles" sensation.

Botn deficiency: low levels of vitamin B7, which is common in pregnant women.

hurosobalamnema: low B2 2 levels

Low levels of Vitamin A are associated with night blindness.

Low prevalence of vitamin C

riskets: severe vitamin D and/or salsium defisiensu

vitamin K defisiensu

Magnesium deficiency occurs with certain medications and medical conditions.

Potassium deficiency is associated with certain medications and health issues.

A balanced diet can aid in preventing these symptoms. Vtamn urrlement mau be necessary for certain roles, such as rregnant or nursing mothers and roles with intrauterine children.

Chapter 3: Common Therapies Your Physician May Prescribe

Before recommending any therapy, including the low-FODMAP diet, your doctor will want to rule out the possibility that you have another significant intestinal disorder with comparable symptoms, such as celiac disease. Your doctor will require a thorough explanation of your problem, including when you first observed symptoms, how frequently they occur, and whether anything in particular triggers or aids in the resolution of your condition.

Your doctor may recommend additional tests, such as blood tests, an upper or lower GI series, ultrasonography, endoscopy, and barium GI studies. A CT scan or an MRI may be necessary for the diagnosis of certain life-threatening conditions. During endoscopic procedures, your physician may perform a biopsy if he or she suspects the presence of other medical issues. In 2 996, the FDA authorized a successful breath test for detecting peptic ulcers without invasive surgery.

If you have a health issue, you may be diagnosed with one of the following conditions:

Inflammatory bowel disease (IBD) Crohn's disease Ulcerative colitis Irritable bowel syndrome (IBS) Acid reflux (GERD) Peptic ulcer

Therapies and management strategies for digestive diseases, such as Crohn's disease and IBS, are tailored to the specific condition and severity of each patient. The fundamental lifestyle modifications are identical to those prescribed for the vast majority of serious medical conditions:

Quit smoking.

Reduce or eliminate your alcohol and caffeine consumption.

Consume small quantities of sustenance.

Get some fresh air and regular exercise.

Utilize meditation or relaxation techniques to unwind.

Heartburn, constipation, and diarrhea can all be remedied with over-the-counter medications. If your symptoms are severe, your doctor may prescribe medication to treat them. Options include fiber supplements, antispasmodics, antacids, and laxatives.

It is difficult in multiple ways to exist within a body that appears to be turning against you. Stress caused by the disease is likely to exacerbate it. Counseling and antidepressants may be required under certain conditions. Surgery may also be used to treat specific conditions, such as enhancing the function of the intestines or reeasily moving bowel obstructions.

A low-FODMAP diet may help many individuals with digestive issues feel better without the really need for medications or their aggravating side effects. Doctors increasingly recommend a low-FODMAP diet to their patients. They may recommend consulting with a dietician or nutritionist because the diet entails a significant change in the meals you prepare and ingest. And this diet is designed to just keep you motivated, as many people report feeling improved soon after beginning it.

The first phase of a FODMAP diet, also known as the elimination phase, is the acute phase. This two-week period is designed to allow your digestive system to acclimate. At this juncture, the objective is to avoid meals that are high in FODMAPs. Fruits, for instance, are limited in the diet, as are portion sizes and consumption frequency. Fresh and preserved fruits, as well as certain vegetables low in FODMAPs, such as sweet potatoes, have recommended serving sizes. This phase is essential for restoring your body's health and feeling good. However, it may be difficult to adhere to a diet that is likely less variegated than what you are used to.

After the acute phase, foods are reintroduced in a controlled succession of "challenges." During this phase, you gradually increase your dietary options by selecting foods and portion sizes that are appropriate for you. Garlic, for example, may be tolerated by some individuals if they do not consume it more than once per day, but it may be problematic for others.

The challenges phase of the diet is structured meticulously over two or three days, with approximately four days between each challenge. Due to this method, you will discover a new world of foods that you previously believed to be problematic are now safe and delicious additions to your diet. It is uncommon for a person who believes they are lactose intolerant to discover that milk is not a trigger item.

On the first day of the challenge, you include approximately half a serving of a high-FODMAP food from the category you're researching. If you experience a mild allergic reaction, you should stop the challenge and revert to the acute phase diet for three or four days before starting the next one. If you do not react to a small portion, attempt a larger amount the next day and observe your reaction. You may safely reintroduce the food to your diet if you can tolerate it, so long as you really do not consume it too frequently or in excessive quantities. Then, you move on to the next challenge, and so on, until you determine which FODMAP foods are acceptable and which are not.

Is brown sugar FODMAP-low?

On our list of limited FODMAP foods, brown sugar is on the FODMAP list. Although brown sugars can be found in many of your beloved dishes, it is prudent to be wary of their various names. Be wary of formulations such as "dextrin," "dextrose," "golden syrup," "maltodextrin," "truffle," and "saccharose," as well as other deceptive names for sweeteners.

Is strawberry FODMAP-free?

Berries are a sustenance of miracles! Numerous studies have disclosed that strawberries are devoid of FODMAP components. As a result, you may be able to consume more strawberries without experiencing IBS symptoms. One serving consists of approximately 2 0 to 2 2 strawberries, or 2 8 0 grams. Upon contact, mature strawberries will feel firm and dense. Be sure to tally your serving size prior to devouring it, as grocery stores and farmer's markets frequently sell them in varying quantities.

What is the better news? Strawberries can be utilized in both sweet and savory dishes. You can consume them on their own, mix them with yogurt, or sprinkle them over your favorite low-FODMAP dish after roasting them.

Strawberry and other low-FODMAP fruits can also be incorporated into homemade granola bars. This strawberry oat bar recipe is excellent. Please use traditional, not instant, cereals! These treats are ideal for daytime travel because they can be prepared in less than an hour in an 8" by 8" baking pan.

Last but not least, pudding has returned to fashion and is a delectable breakfast treat or afternoon snack. This Monash University recipe is a quick and easy method to incorporate strawberries into your diet, as they are a low FODMAP fruit. This pudding, which has been sweetened with maple syrup, is another example of how you can enjoy delicious food without becoming unwell.

Is Sushi FODMAP-free?

Sushi may be a safe option. On a low-FODMAP diet, soy sauce's trace concentrations of gluten are typically not a problem. If avocado is included in your sushi rolls, you must limit your consumption. Due to the wheat content of tempura rolls, you may want to avoid them or consume only one during the elimination phase. Both rice and seaweed contain naturally minimal levels of FODMAPs.

Chapter 4: Follow These Three Measures Prior To Beginning A Low-Fodmap Diet.

2 . Ensure that you have IBS digestive symptoms in multiple instances, some of which are harmful and others more significant. IBS symptoms are also common in conditions such as celiac disease, inflammatory bowel disease, defecation disorders, and colon cancer. Therefore, you should consult a physician to rule out these other possibilities. Once these have been ruled out, your physician can corroborate that you have IBS using an off-the-shelf diagnostic test. To be diagnosed with IBS, you must satisfy all three of the criteria listed below.

Recurrent abdominal ran. In the past three months, your pain has occurred at least once per week on average.

Stool sumrtoms. Thee should satisfy at least two of the following: related to decline, associated with a change in tool frequency, or associated with a change in tool distribution.

Persistent sumrtoms. You have experienced persistent symptoms for the past three months, with symptom onset occurring at least six months prior to diagnosis.

2. Consider lifestyle and dietary modification techniques

The low FODMAP diet is both time- and resource-intensive. This is still considered second-line treatment advice in some countries and is only used to treat IBS. who do not respond to initial strategies.

6 . Prepare ahead

It may be difficult to adhere to the low FODMAP diet's restrictions. Here are some suggestions to assist you in preparing:

Determine what to buy. Ensure you have access to an acceptable low FODMAP food list. Eliminate high FODMAP foods. Clear your refrigerator and larder of these items to avoid making a mistake. Create a horrifying lt. Create a low FODMAP shopping list before heading to the supermarket so you know which foods to purchase and which to avoid. Consult menus in advance. Familiarize yourself with low FODMAP menu options so you can dine out with confidence. Garlic and onions are high in FODMAPs. This has contributed to the widespread misconception that a low FODMAP diet is flavorless. While many recipes call for onion and garlic, you can choose from a variety of low FODMAP herbs, spices, and seasonings.

In addition, you can obtain the flavor of garlic by using garlic-infused oil that is low in FODMAPs. This is because the FODMAPs in garlic are not fat-soluble, so only the garlic flavor is conveyed to the oil.

Singapore Noodles

Ingredients:

- 1/2 cup of chopped scallions
- 1/2 cup of chopped cilantro
- 2 lime, juiced
- sriracha sauce, to taste

- 2 lb. of firm tofu
- 2 tbsp. soy sauce
- 2 tbsp. vegetable oil
- 16 oz. of angel hair pasta

Instructions:

1. Preheat your oven to 350 degrees Fahrenheit.

2. Cut the tofu into small cubes and toss with soy sauce and vegetable oil.

3. Spread the tofu onto a baking sheet and roast for 25-30 minutes, or until golden brown and easy cook ed through.

4. Easy cook the angel hair pasta in a large pot of boiling water according to package instructions, or until al dente.

5. Drain the pasta and return it to the pot. Add the roasted tofu, scallions, cilantro, lime juice, sriracha sauce, and salt and pepper to taste.

6. Toss to combine and serve hot!

Wasabi-Toasted Nori Croissant

Ingredients

4 tablespoons powdered horseradish wasabi
20 sheets nori
1/2 cup water
salt

Instructions

1. Heat oven to 250°F.
2. Combine the water and the wasabi in a small bowl and whisk with a fork until the wasabi is dissolved.
3. The wasabi tends to settle to the bottom, so you may really need to re-whisk between batches.

Low-Fodmap Vegetable Risotto

Ingredients

250 ml/10 fl oz dry white wine
400g/7oz spinach leaves
10 0g/2 ¾oz Parmesan cheese grated
2 tsp flaked sea salt and freshly ground black pepper
6 tbsp garlic infused oil
250 g/10 oz butternut squash, peeled, deseeded and cut into roughly
6 cm/2 ¼in chunks
2 tsp yeast extract
1 tsp dried mixed herbs
2 celery stick, finely chopped
600 g/2 0½oz risotto rice
6 carrots (around 6 00g/2 0½oz), peeled and coarsely grated

Method

1. Heat 2   tablespoon of the oil in a medium frying pan over a low–

medium heat and fry the squash for 20 minutes, until tender and lightly browned, turning regularly.

2. Pour 2 .2 litres/2 pints of water into a large saucepan and add the yeast extract, herbs and salt.

3. Bring to a gentle simmer to make a quick stock, stirring occasionally.

4. Leave to stand.

5. While the squash is cooking, heat the remaining oil in a large, saucepan and fry the celery for 1-5 minutes, stirring.

6. Add the rice and easy cook for 1-5 minute more.

7. Stir in the wine and simmer until it has almost disappeared.

8. Stir in the grated carrots and easy cook for a few seconds.

9. Add a ladleful of the warm stock to the pan and easy cook , stirring regularly, until it has been absorbed by the rice .

10. Continue adding the stock, stirring well between each addition.
11. Cook, until the rice is tender and the sauce is creamy.
12. This will take 35 to 40 minutes.
13. Add two thirds of the Parmesan and spinach leaves, a handful at a time, and easy cook until the leaves are soft and the cheese has melted.
14. Season with salt and pepper and stir in half the easy cook ed squash.
15. Spoon into serving dishes and top with the remaining squash.
16. Sprinkle with the rest of the cheese and serve immediately.

Chicken Parmesan With Low Fodmap

easy cook easy cook

Two-Pepper Cornbread

Ingredients:

- 2 tablespoon melted butter
- 4 tablespoons diced red onion
- 2 tablespoon diced green bell pepper
- 2 tablespoon diced yellow bell pepper

- 2 cup all-purpose flour
- 2 teaspoon baking powder
- 1 teaspoon baking soda
- 1/2 teaspoon ground black pepper
- 1/2 teaspoon salt
- 1 cup buttermilk

Directions:

1. Preheat oven to 450 degrees F (200 degrees C). Grease a 9x2 6 inch baking dish.

2. In a medium bowl, combine flour, baking powder, baking soda and pepper; set aside.
3. In another medium bowl, whisk buttermilk and melted butter.
4. Pour buttermilk mixture into the flour mixture; mix well.
5. Stir in red onion, green bell pepper, yellow bell pepper and 1-5 tablespoon of cheese.
6. Bake for 35 to 40 minutes or until bread is golden brown.

Macaroni With Cheese

INGREDIENTS

- 1 tsp. pepper
- 2 1 cups milk
- ¼ pound thinly sliced cheddar cheese
- 8 Tbsp. butter
- 2 large onion, finely chopped
- 8 cups easy cook ed macaroni
- 2 tsp. salt

PREPARATIONS

1. Melt butter in a frying pan, then fry onion over medium heat for 24 minutes.
2. Stir in remaining ingredients, except cheese, then transfer frying pan contents to a greased casserole.

3. Top evenly with cheese and bake uncovered in a 350° F preheated oven for 80 minutes.
4. Serve from the casserole while warm.

Low Fodmar Ntant Rot Chunky Salsa

INGREDIENTS

- 6 cups fresh common tomatoes*and their juices or 28 ounce can diced tomatoes and their juices
- 1 cup scallions, dark green parts only, chopped
- 2 tablespoon dried chives
- 2 1 teaspoons ground cumin
- 2 1 teaspoons salt
- 1 teaspoon pepper
- 4 tablespoons garlic-infused olive oil
- 2 1 cups green bell pepper, diced
- 1 cup jalapeño peppers, seeds removed, diced • 1 cup leek, green tops only, finely-chopped
- 2 teaspoon red pepper flakes
- 1 cup water

• ½ cup white vinegar • 6 tablespoons lime juice, freshly squeezed

INSTRUCTIONS

1. Prepare ingredients: Prepare all ingredients per the list above before starting to cook.
2. Sauté: Hit the "Sauté" button on your 12-quart Instant Pot, 16-quart Instant Pot, or comparable electric pressure easy cook er.
3. Once the display reads "Hot," add garlic-infused olive oil and swirl the Instant Pot to coat the bottom in oil.
4. Add green pepper, jalapeno, and leeks and sauté for 5-10 minutes, stirring frequently.
5. Add red pepper flakes and sauté for 60 seconds, stirring constantly. Hit "Cancel" on the Instant Pot.
6. Add liquids and seasonings: Pour in water, vinegar, and lime juice and scrape the bottom of the pot clean with a plastic spoon if needed.

7. Add tomatoes and their juices, scallions, dried chives, cumin, salt, and pepper and stir until combined.

8. Pressure cook: Close the Instant Pot, set the pressure release valve to "Sealing" hit the "Pressure Cook" or "Manual" button, and set the timer for 5-10 minutes.

9. Turn the "Keep Warm" button off.

10. Naturally release pressure: Once the cooking cycle has completed, allow the pressure to release naturally for 20 minutes, and then manually release the remaining pressure.

11. Just cool and refrigerate: Open lid and stir salsa. Allow to cool in the Instant Pot, uncovered, for 2 0 minutes.

12. Transfer to an airtight container and refrigerate for a minimum of 8 hours prior to eating.

13. Stir, taste, and adjust seasonings, vinegar and/or lime juice as desired (see notes).
14. Serve: serve with my upcoming Low FODMAP Instant Pot Salsa Chicken, as a topping on my Low FODMAP Instant Pot Carnitas, Low FODMAP Wet Burrito Bowls, low FODMAP tacos, nachos, or as a snack with compliant tortilla chips.

Fodmar, Leek, And Rotato Our Served With Bason.

INGREDIENTS

- 6 cups low FODMAP chicken bone broth
- 2 tablespoon dried chives
- 2 1 teaspoons sea salt
- 1 teaspoon ground black pepper
- 1 teaspoon dried thyme or
1 tablespoon fresh thyme leaves
- 1 teaspoon smoked paprika
- 1 cup coconut cream**
- 12 strips nitrate-free, sugar-free, low sodium bacon, cut into ½-inch pieces
- 4 tablespoons garlic-infused olive oil
- 2 1 cups leek, dark green leaves only, thinly sliced*

- 4 pounds red potatoes peeled or unpeeled, chopped into 2 -inch pieces

INSTRUCTIONS

1. Sauté bacon: Hit "Sauté" on your 12-quart Instant Pot, 16-quart Instant Pot, or comparable electric pressure easy cook er.
2. Add chopped bacon to the pot, and sauté until crisp, about 15 minutes.
3. Using a slotted spoon, remove bacon pieces to a plate covered in paper towel, leaving the bacon fat in the pot.
4. Set bacon aside.
5. Sauté leeks: Add garlic-infused oil to the pot and swirl to coat.
6. Add leeks and sauté for 5-10 minutes, stirring frequently.
7. Add broth and scrape: Hit "Cancel" on the Instant Pot.

8. Add 2 cup of the chicken bone broth, wait about 2 10 seconds, and scrape the bottom of the pot clean with a plastic spoon.

9. Add the remaining 2 cups of broth.

10. Add herbs and spices: Add dried chives, salt, pepper, thyme, and smoked paprika to the pot and stir.

11. Add chopped potatoes and stir again to distribute evenly in the broth.

12. Pressure cook: Close the lid and set the pressure release valve to "Sealing."

13. Press the "Pressure Cook" button and set the timer for 20 minutes.

14. Blend: Once the easy cook ing cycle has completed, quick release the pressure.

15. Open lid and allow the soup to cool for a few minutes.

16. Using an immersion blender, carefully blend the soup to your

desired consistency, leaving some of the soup chunky or blending the soup until just smooth (do not over-blend).

17. Add remaining ingredients: Add coconut cream and ⅔ of the reserved bacon to the soup and stir.

18. Taste the soup and adjust seasonings as desired.

19. Chop the remaining ⅓ of the bacon into small pieces.

20. Garnish with the chopped bacon, fresh chopped chives and/or freshly ground black pepper (optional). Serve and enjoy.

Individual Strawberru & Rhubarb Quinoa Srumbles

Ingredients

900 g quinoa flakes

130 g walnuts, chopped

4 tsp cinnamon

6 tbsp coconut oil, melted

2 tsp pure vanilla extract

400g rhubarb

800g strawberries, hulled

Juice of 1 a lime

12 tbsp maple syrup

250 g gluten-free oats

2 tbsp brown sugar to top (optional)

Lactose-free cream to serve (optional)

Ingredients

1. Preheat the oven to 200°C (gas 8). Grease individual tins or ramekins

with a little coconut oil and put to one side.

2. Chop the rhubarb, slice the strawberries, and place in a large bowl.

3. Add the lime juice and 4 tablespoons of the maple syrup and stir to combine.

4. Divide the fruit among the ramekins.

5. To make the crumble, put the oats, quinoa flakes, walnuts and cinnamon in a large bowl and stir to combine.

6. Add the coconut oil, remaining 5-10 tablespoons of maple syrup and vanilla extract and stir once more.

7. Spoon the crumble mixture on top of the fruit in each dish and sprinkle with a little brown sugar if desired.

8. Bake for 45-50 minutes, or until the crumble is golden brown and the fruit is bubbling.

9. Serve warm with a generous dollop of lactose-free cream.

8. French Toast With Bananas

Ingredients

For The Bread:
grams

- 1 cup coconut flour, 10 6 grams

- 1/2 teaspoon sea salt

French Toast
- 4 eggs
- 1 teaspoon cinnamon

- 1/2 cup almond milk, 60 ml, or dairy free milk of your choice

- 2 teaspoon vanilla extract

- coconut oil for frying

- 2 teaspoon cinnamon

- 8 eggs
- 2 teaspoon vanilla extract

- 4 mashed ripe bananas-the darker/spottier, the better

- 2 teaspoon baking soda

- 1-5 cup maple syrup or honey, 80 grams, maple for low FODMAP

- 1 cup melted coconut oil, 2 010 grams, or butter/ ghee

- 1 cup almond flour, 100

Instructions

For The Bread

1. Set the oven to 350°F/200°C.
2. In a bowl of medium size, beat the eggs.
3. Next add the butter or oil, vanilla, and maple syrup to the eggs and mix thoroughly.
4. Combine the remaining wet ingredients with the mashed bananas.

5. In a small bowl, combine the dry ingredients while sifting to get rid of any clumps.
6. Mix the dry ingredients thoroughly after adding them to the liquid, do this until it is smooth.
7. You can do this by hand, but I found that an electric mixer produced a batter that was smoother.
8. Scoop your batter into the loaf pan after greasing or lining it with parchment paper. set aside.
9. Bake in the oven for 80 to 90 minutes, or until a knife inserted in the center easy come out clean.
10. Before using the banana bread to easy make French toast, let it cool completely.
11. Leave it alone over night if possible.

For the French toast

1. Slice your banana bread into pieces that are 2 inch thick.
2. Next Grease a skillet or griddle pan with oil after heating it over medium heat.
3. Whisk the eggs, milk, vanilla, and cinnamon together in a shallow bowl.
4. Slices of banana bread should be dipped into the egg mixture one at a time.
5. After coating both sides of the bread, place it in the skillet and easy cook the first side until it is just beginning to turn slightly crispy.
6. Each side should just take two to three minutes.
7. Continue until done, then top with extra banana slices, drizzle more chocolate if you're feeling particularly indulgent, and if you'd like, whipped cream.

Cardamom Rice Pudding

Instructions

choice

40g lactose-free butter, plus extra for greasing

Toasted coconut, to serve

250 g pudding rice

20 cardamom pods, lightly crushed

100 g brown sugar

2 litre lactose- or dairy-free milk of

Instructions

1. Preheat the oven to 250 °C (gas 2) and lightly butter a 10 litre ovenproof dish.
2. Into the dish toss the rice, cardamom pods and sugar.
3. Stir in the milk, dot with the butter and put in the oven.

4. Cook the pudding for 60 minutes then give it a stir.
5. Return to the oven for a further 60 minutes before stirring again.
6. Return to the oven for a final hour; by this time the rice should be tender and creamy.
7. Serve hot with a handful of toasted nuts or coconut.

Beef Stock

Ingredients:

- 4 bay leaves
- 2 0 black peppercorns
- 6 quarts cold water

- 2 lb. beef bones
- 2 onion, chopped
- 8 carrots, chopped
- 8 celery stalks, chopped

Instructions:

1. In a large pot or Dutch oven, combine the beef bones, onion, carrots, celery and bay leaves.
2. Cover with cold water and bring to a boil over high heat.

3. Reduce the heat to low and simmer for 6 hours.
4. Strain the stock through a fine mesh strainer into a clean pot.
5. Discard the bones and vegetables.
6. Bring the stock to a simmer over medium heat and season with salt and pepper to taste.
7. Serve hot or cold.

Citrus-Flavored Overnight Oatmeal

Ingredients:

- ½ teaspoon cinnamon
- 1 teaspoon vanilla extract
- ½ teaspoon orange extract
- 1/7 teaspoon ground ginger
- 2 cup gluten-free rolled oats
- 3 cups lactose-free milk, divided
- Juice of 1 orange
- 1 tablespoon chia seeds
- 2 tablespoon maple syrup, divided

Directions:

1. In a medium bowl, stir together the oats, 2 cup of the milk, orange juice, chia seeds, half of the maple syrup, cinnamon, vanilla and orange extracts, and ginger.
2. Cover and refrigerate overnight.

3. To serve, stir in the remaining maple syrup, and serve chilled or warmed.

Coconut-Pineapple Smoothie

Ingredients:

- 2 cup unsweetened almond milk
- 2 cup crushed ice
- 4 tablespoons chia seeds or flaxseed
- 4 cups crushed pineapple, fresh or canned in water and drained
- 2 cup canned full-fat coconut milk

Directions:

1. In a blender, combine the pineapple, coconut milk, almond milk, ice, and chia seeds.
2. Blend until smooth.

Vanilla Flavored Oats

Ingredients:

- tablespoons coconut sugar
- 2 teaspoon espresso powder
- 4 teaspoons vanilla extract

- cup almond milk
- and 1 cups of water
- cup old fashioned oats

Instruction:

1. Add milk, oats, sugar, espresso, vanilla extract to your Instant Pot and toss.

2. Close lid and easy cook on HIGH pressure for 20 minutes.

3. Release pressure naturally over 20 minutes.

4. Stir and divide into serving bowls. Serve and enjoy!

Bacon-Jalapeño Egg Cups

Ingredients:

For the Bacon

tablespoon butter

12 bacon slices
For the Eggs

- ½ cup shredded Mexican blend cheese
- 4 ounces cream cheese, at room temperature

- jalapeño peppers
- 8 large eggs
- Pink Himalayan salt
- Freshly ground black pepper

Instruction:

1. Preheat the oven to 350 °F. While the oven is warming up, heat a large skillet over medium-high heat.

2. Add the bacon slices and easy cook partially, about 5-10 minutes.

3. Transfer the bacon to a paper towel–lined plate.

4. Coat six cups of a standard muffin tin with the butter.

5. Place a partially cooked bacon strip in each cup to line the sides.

6. To make the Eggs: Cut one jalapeño lengthwise, seed it, and mince it.

7. Cut the remaining jalapeño into rings, discarding the seeds.

8. Set aside. In a medium bowl, beat the fresh eggs with a hand mixer until well beaten.

9. Add the cream cheese and diced jalapeño, season with pink.

10. Himalayan salt and pepper, and beat again to combine.

11. Pour the egg mixture into the prepared muffin tin, filling each cup about two-thirds of the way up so they have room to rise.

12. Top each cup with some of the shredded cheese and a ring of jalapeño, and bake for 35-40 minutes.

13. Just cool for 2 0 minutes, and serve hot.

Buckwheat Muffins

INGREDIENTS

- 2 tbsp apple cider vinegar or white vinegar
- 4 cups light buckwheat flour
- 4 tsp baking powder
- ½ tsp salt
- 1 cup dairy-free chocolate chips
- 2 cup grated carrot
- 2 medium ripe banana
- ½ cup almond butter
- 1 cup monk fruit sweetener for sugar-free or coconut sugar
- 1/2 cup plant-based milk such as unsweetened almond milk

Directions

1. Preheat the oven to 350 degrees F.

2. Using a fork or immersion blender, mash the banana into a paste in a large mixing bowl.

3. Add the almond butter, milk, sugar and vinegar and mix until completely smooth and creamy.

4. Add the buckwheat flour, baking powder and salt.

5. While they're sitting on top of the wet ingredients, gently mix the dry ingredients together to incorporate the baking powder and salt, then fold the dry ingredients into the wet until all the flour is wetted.

6. Do not overmix the batter.

7. Fold it just enough to wet all the flour, then stop mixing.

8. Add the chocolate chips and grated carrot and gently fold them in a few times to mix.

9. Spray a standard-size muffin pan with a light coating of non-stick cooking spray. Evenly divide the batter between 15-20 muffin cups.

10. Bake for 35-40 minutes until browned and firm on top.

11. Remove from the oven and let cool in the pan for 8 -10 minutes then gently pop them out using a knife and place them on a cooling rack.

12. Let cool completely before storing or enjoy warm with vegan butter.

13. Store the muffins in an airtight container at room temperature for up

to 6 days, in the fridge for up to 2 week or freeze for up to 6 months

Banana Porridge

4 bananas, one mashed and one sliced

4 tablespoon ground almonds

4 tablespoon honey

200 g rolled oats

1400 ml semi-skimmed milk

HOW TO EASY MAKE

tir together the oats, mashed banana, almonds, and milk in a saucepan.

To start, bring water to a boil. It's then time to turn the heat down to low and easy cook the food for about 8 to 10 minutes, often stirring

so it doesn't stick to the bottom.

When you're done, divide the mixture into two bowls and top each one with honey, banana slices, and other things you want.

Courgette Pasta With Pine Nuts Low In Fodmaps

Ingredients:

10 anchovy fillets

 2 tablespoon of garlic-implanted olive oil in addition to some extra to complete

A little spot of dried bean stew flakes

 Grated parmesan cheese

 A touch of ground dark pepper 380 grams sans gluten pasta

 2 medium-sized courgette, cut into short sticks A

 modest bunch of pine nuts

Procedure:

1. Easy cook pasta in a huge pot of bubbling water.
2. Easy cook as indicated by bundle guidelines, until still somewhat firm.
3. Mix sometimes while easy cook ing to just keep the pasta from adhering to the base.
4. Channel when easy cook ed however saved 100 ml of the easy cook ing water.
5. Heat skillet over medium hotness settings.
6. Gently toast pine nuts with next to no additional oils.
7. Throw until the nuts begin to brown and become fragrant.
8. Eliminate from the container and set aside.
9. In a similar dish, add garlic-mixed olive oil.
10. Add the anchovy filets advertisement the stew drops.

11. Separate the anchovies with a wooden spoon and fry for a couple minutes.

12. Add courgette and pan fried food until it begins to mellow.

13. Transform off the heat. Add the easy cook ed pasta into the dish.

14. Add saved pasta easy cook ing water and a big part of the parmesan cheddar.

15. Throw to blend all that together.

16. Serve by fixing with pine nuts and remaining parmesan cheddar.

17. Shower a modest quantity of garlic-mixed olive oil.

Smoothie Of Bananas And Vegetables

Ingredients:

- 2 apple, cored, peeled, and cut up

- 2 pear, cored, peeled, and cut up 2 cups water

- **2 banana, cut up**
- 4 cups baby spinach, chopped

Instructions:

1. In a blender or with a strong hand blender, combine all the ingredients.
2. After blending until smooth, serve.

Garlic -Infused Olive Oil

INGREDIENTS

- 2 cup plus 2 tsp. extra-virgin olive oil
- 16 garlic cloves

Directions:

1. In a small, heavy saucepan, boil the oil and garlic over medium heat until the garlic begins to crackle and little bubbles rise steadily to the top.

2. Easy cook for 20 minutes, or until the garlic is tender, over low heat.

3. After letting it cool for a little while, just take out the garlic and carefully lock the oil in the refrigerator to just keep it fresh for up to 1-5 days.

Coconut Oat Granola

Ingredients:

- 2 tsp rosewater
- 2 tsp vanilla concentrate
- 200g dull chocolate, broken into pieces
- Almond or other milk, to serve
- Eatable blossoms or new organic product
- 180g oats, mixed into flour
- 180g destroyed coconut
- 160 ml coconut oil, fluid
- 120 ml maple syrup
- 1/7 tsp ocean salt
- 2 tin (8 00ml) full-fat coconut milk

Directions:

1. Preheat stove to 200ºC/350ºF/Gas Mark 8.

2. To easy make the hull, consolidate coconut oil, maple syrup, oat flour and destroyed coconut together in a blending bowl.

3. Oil a little preparing tin with coconut oil and press blend into the base before putting into the broiler and easy cook for 35-40 minutes until fresh.

4. Expel from the broiler and put aside to cool and solidify.

5. In the meantime, scoop out the strong coconut cream from the tin and into a huge bowl.

6. Quit scooping when you arrive at the water in the base of the can.

7. Utilizing a blender or hand mixers on rapid – whip the coconut cream for 5-10 minutes until it gets cushioned and light, with delicate pinnacles.

8. Mix through the vanilla and rosewater.

9. When the granola has easy cook ed and cooled, separate into lumps and partition crosswise over bowls.

10. Top with rosewater cream, dull chocolate and eatable blossoms or new organic product.

11. Present with your preferred lactose-or without dairy milk.

Salsa Verde

INGREDIENTS

- 2 tbsp. garlic-infused olive oil
- 4 tbsp. olive oil
- 4 tbsp. fresh lemon juice, or to taste
- Salt and freshly ground black pepper
- 4 handfuls of flat-leaf parsley, rinsed and dried
- 6 anchovy fillets in oil, drained (optional)
- 4 tsp. capers, rinsed and drained

Directions:

1. The parsley, capers, and anchovy fillets (if using) should be combined in a food processor or blender and blended until smooth.

2. Drizzle the olive oil and garlic-infused oil in small amounts, thoroughly combining after each addition.

3. Add the lemon juice and season with salt and pepper to taste.

4. Place in a dish or jar, cover, and refrigerate for up to 10 days.

Pickled Carrots

- 4 teaspoons sea salt
- ½ teaspoon red pepper flakes
- 2 pound baby carrots or carrots cut into sticks
- 6 cups water, plus more as needed
- 2 cup red wine vinegar

1. Combine the water, vinegar, salt, and red pepper flakes in a large bowl or a glass jar.
2. Stir until the salt dissolves.
3. Add the carrots to the bowl.
4. Add more water if necessary to completely submerge the carrots.
5. 2.Marinate in the refrigerator for at least 20 to 24 hours and up to 8 days before serving.

Fresh Spring Rolls Made By Hand

Ingredients:

- 4 cups of destroyed romaine lettuce
- 2 scallion, green and white parts, slashed
- 2 bundle of cilantro, slashed
- sauce of decision, I prescribe Thai Peanut Sauce
- 24 rice paper spring move wrappers
- 4 huge carrots, stripped and cut julienne style
- 2 little zucchini as well as cucumber, cut julienne style
- 2 chime pepper, any shading, cut julienne style
- 2 cup destroyed red cabbage
- 2 avocado, cut meager

Directions:

1. Before beginning, gently wet your work surface just keep .

2. Just take a solitary dry rice spring move wrapper and spot it in the bowl of tepid warm water.

3. Give the rice a chance to paper sit in the water for 50 seconds, or until it gets flexible.

4. This is the crucial step: just keep on feeling how adaptable the rice paper is.

5. You really need it to be delicate and functional without being soft.

6. At the point when you feel like the rice paper is prepared, remove the spring move wrapper from the water and lay it down a level on your wet surface.

7. You will really need to work rapidly from here.

8. Beginning in the focal point of the wrapper, place the carrot, zucchini and ringer pepper cuts in a rectangular shape, avoiding the edges of the wrapper.

9. Just keep on including the entirety of the fillings, from the purple cabbage to the cilantro, by setting everything in the inside, individually, keeping up the square shape in the center.

10.   Work rapidly; you really do not really need your wrapper to self-destruct.

11.   At the point when you've set the entirety of your fixings in a decent heap in the spring move wrapper, it's a great opportunity to move it shut!

12.   Note: Be mindful so as not to overload your spring move wrapper

since it will cause the rice paper to tear and start by collapsing the top and base segments of the rice paper in over the vegetables.

13.   Beginning the left-hand side, stretch the left half of the wrapper around the heap of recipes, tucking and easily moving until you can rest the wrapper simply under the fixings.

14.   Just take care of the corners and afterwards just keep on rolling the spring moves the whole distance, making your move as tight as conceivable without tearing the rice paper wrapper.

15.   That is, it, and you simply rolled your own special spring roll! Presently, move the same number of spring moves as you might want and appreciate immediately.

16.   Appreciate your most loved plunging sauce.

17.   I prescribe a Thai Peanut Sauce, anything with Ginger, Soy Sauce or Coconut Aminos!

Low Fodmap Alaskan Salmon Chowder

INGREDIENTS:

- pound (8 10 10   g) Yukon gold potatoes, peeled and cut into large dice
- 6   medium carrots, trimmed, peeled and cut crosswise into ½-inch rounds
- 2 bay leaf
- 1 teaspoon dried thyme
- pound (8 10 10   g) skinned salmon, preferably Atlantic, cut into large chunks
- Kosher salt
- Freshly ground black pepper
- 4 tablespoons Low FODMAP Onion-Infused Oil or extra-virgin olive oil
- 2 cup (68 g) chopped scallions, green parts only

- 1 cup (6 6 g) finely chopped leeks, green parts only
- 8 cups (960 ml) UHT unsweetened coconut milk
- 4 cups (8 80 ml) low FODMAP stock – fish (clam) or chicken
- pound (8 10 10 g) celeriac, peeled and cut into large dice

PREPARATION:

1. Heat oil in a large soup pot or Dutch oven over low-medium heat until shimmering.
2. Add scallion and leek greens and sauté until softened but not browned, just a few minutes, then add coconut milk, stock, celeriac and potato dice, carrots, bay leaf and thyme and stir everything together well.
3. Bring to a simmer and easy cook until celeriac and potatoes are tender, about 20 minutes.
4. Add the fish and continue to simmer until fish is opaque and easy cook ed through; this will be about 10 minutes.
5. Taste and season with salt and pepper; serve immediately.

Pad Thai Noodles

INGREDIENTS:

200g beansprouts end trimmed
4 tablespoons peanuts, chopped coarsely
Lime wedges, for garnish
500 g rice stick noodles
4 tablespoons Rice Oil
4 eggs, scrambled a bit
• 1/2 cup pad Thai paste
500g firm tofu, chopped into fine pieces

DIRECTIONS:

1. Add the rice noodles in a heatproof bowl. Cover w/ boiling hot water.
2. Stand for 20 minutes until softened. Drain the noodles in a colander.
3. Set the noodles aside.
4. Heat 2 Tsp. Of oil in a large frying pan.

5. Add egg and fry softly enough that the white is set.
6. Easy cook for 1-5 minutes and remove to a plate.
7. Roughly chop the egg.
8. Heat the remaining oil in the pan. Add the Thai paste and tofu.
9. Stir together in the oil for 2 minute or until fragrant.
10. Add the rice noodles.
11. Cook, stirring, for 2 minute or until the noodles are warmed. Remove from heat.
12. Divide the noodle mixture between the serving bowls.
13. Place the beansprouts on top, then the pieces of egg, then the peanuts.
14. Squirt a spritz of lime juice into the noodles and serve with decorative lime pieces.

Sea Bass With Citrus

Ingredients

- 2 tbsp olive oil
- 8 x 600g whole small sea bass, scaled, gutted and slashed a few times down each side
- 5-10 large oranges
- zest 2 lemon (use the juice below)

For the salad
- 4 bags watercress
- handful small capers
- handful pitted green olives, roughly chopped

- 4 oranges, segmented
- juice 2 lemon
- 8 tbsp olive oil

Method

1. Finely grate the zest of 2 of the oranges and add to the lemon zest.
2. Mix with the olive oil, then drizzle over the fish and season.
3. Cut the rest of the oranges into slices about 10 mm thick.
4. When the coals are ashen, arrange the orange slices over the barbecue in groups the length of each fish.
5. Char the orange slices on 2 side, then flip them over and lay the fish on top of them – this stops the fish sticking.
6. Barbecue the fish for 10-15 mins on each side or until the flesh flakes away easily when prodded.
7. While the fish is barbecuing easy make the salad.
8. Put the orange segments in a large bowl with the squeezed juice from

the rest of the oranges and the lemon juice.

9. Season and stir in the olive oil.

10. When the fish is easy cook ed, toss the watercress in the orange dressing with the capers and olives.

11. Serve the fish with the salad.

Broccoli Tahini Soup

- 400ml /7fl oz cant 2 cup vegetable stock seasoned with salt and pepper
- Topping 25-30 g tahini
- 0100 g coconut yogurt
- 2 tbsp lemon juice
- 2 tablespoon of chopped cilantro coriander leaves
- 2 tbsp olive oil or avocado oil
- 2 minced small onion 2 crushed garlic cloves
- optional 2 tablespoon nutritional yeast flakes
- 2 cm/0.10 in of ginger root, peeled and grated
- 600g broccoli, cut into florets
- 800g/2 8 oz can of coconut milk

1. Cook the onion, garlic, and ginger in a large saucepan over medium heat for

5-10 minutes, or until the onion begins to soften.

2. Add the broccoli, leek, milk, yeast granules, and vegetable stock to the pan. Bring to a boil, then reduce heat and simmer until broccoli is tender, approximately 1-5 minutes.

3. season with salt and pepper to flavor.

4. Combine the tahini, yogurt, and lemon juice with 1-5 tablespoons of water until a viscous sauce forms.

5. Pour the soup into bowls, swirl in the tahini cream, and garnish with coriander cilantro fronds before serving.

Mild And Creamu Butterless Butter Chisken

Ingredients

2 cup full-fat coconut milk

1 cup Low-FODMAP Basic Chicken Bone Broth (here)

4 tablespoons freshly squeezed lemon juice (from 1 lemon)

2 teaspoon sea salt

4 pounds boneless, skinless chicken thighs, cut into 2-inch pieces

½ cup roughly chopped fresh cilantro leaves

½ cup grass-fed ghee or coconut oil

2 tablespoon ground turmeric

4 teaspoons ground cumin

2 teaspoon garam masala

4 tablespoons minced fresh ginger

4 tablespoons tomato paste

Instructions

1. In a large, lidded saucepan, heat the ghee or oil over medium-low heat.
2. Add the turmeric, cumin, garam masala, ginger, and tomato paste.
3. Cook for 1-5 minutes, or until a fragrant paste forms.

4. Carefully stir in the coconut milk, broth, lemon juice, and salt.

5. Bring the sauce to a simmer and easy cook over medium-low heat until slightly reduced and golden in hue, 2 0 minutes.

6. Fold in the chicken and continue to simmer over medium heat, stirring occasionally, for 20 minutes.

7. Place the lid on the pan and simmer for another 15-20 minutes, or until the chicken is tender enough to break apart with your spatula.

8. Serve immediately with the cilantro as garnish.

A Salad Of Chicken And Grapes

2 2 ounces boneless, skinless chicken breast, grilled and cut into ½-inch cubes

6 chopped celery stalks

chopped fennel, 1 cup

Half a cup of green grapes

Chopped walnuts, 1 cup

2 cup of low-FODMAP mayo

One-half teaspoon each of sea salt

1 half teaspoon each of sea salt 8 big leaves of butter lettuce

1. Combine the chicken, celery, fennel, green grapes, and walnuts in a big bowl by tossing everything together.
2. Add the salt, pepper, and mayonnaise. To blend, toss once more.
3. Butter lettuce leaves should be used to serve the salad.

4. Coconut cubes

Gluten-Free Pumpkin Swirl Bread with Cream Cheese Glaze from Fodu'.

Ingredients:

1 tsp ground cardamom

1 tsp salt

4 large fresh eggs

230 oz can pumpkin puree ½ cup maple syrup

2 tsp vanilla extract

½ cup almond milk

4 oz cream cheese, softened 2 cup powdered sugar

2 tsp vanilla extract

6 tbsp almond milk

4 cups gluten-free 2 :2 flour 2 tsp baking powder

2 tsp baking soda

6 tsp ground cinnamon

2 tsp ground nutmeg

2 tsp ground ginger

1 tsp ground clove

Directions

1. Pre-heat oven to 350 0F and grease + line a loaf pan with parchment paper.
2. In a medium mixing bowl, combine gluten-free flour, baking powder, baking soda, salt and spices, mixing gently with a fork to fully incorporate.
3. In a separate large mixing bowl, beat eggs. Next, whisk in pumpkin puree, maple syrup, vanilla and milk continuing to whisk until fully combined.
4. Fold dry ingredients into wet using a silicone spatula + continue mixing until batter is smooth and all dry ingredients are incorporated.
5. Pour batter into loaf pan and bake for 80 to 90 minutes or until a toothpick comes out clean.
6. While pumpkin spice loaf is baking, prepare the cream cheese glaze in a small bowl.

7. Using a silicone spatula, continue to soften cream cheese until smooth.

8. Gradually add powdered sugar, milk, and vanilla, whisking gently until smooth.

9. Alternatively, this can be done using a hand mixer or stand mixer.

10. Once loaf is finished baking, allow to cool at room temperature for 20 minutes before topping with glaze.

11. Serve your pumpkin spice loaf warm and enjoy!

Salmon With Salsa Verde

Ingredients

- 4 lemons, juice only
- 8 salmon fillets
- To serve (optional)
- 250 g wild and white basmati rice
- 100 g stoned marinated black kalamata olive
- 150 g toasted pine nut
- 2 red pepper, chopped

- 2 x 210 g pack dill, roughly chopped
- 2 x 210 g pack mint, tough stalks removed and roughly chopped
- 2 x 210 g pack flat-leaf parsley, roughly chopped
- 2 x 210 g pack chives, roughly chopped
- 2 1 tbsp wholegrain mustard
- 4 tbsp caper
- 4 tbsp toasted pine nut
- 2 x 200g tin green olive stuffed with anchovies, drained (810 g)

Method

- Preheat the oven to 250C/fan 2 80C/gas 6. To easy make the salsa verde, put the herbs, mustard, capers, pine nuts, olives and the juice of the 2 1 lemons in a food processor and pulse until roughly chopped.
- Put the salmon fillets on a lightly oiled baking sheet.
- Squeeze over the juice of the remaining half lemon and season with freshly ground black pepper.
- Easy cook in the oven for 10 to 15 minutes or until easy cook ed through.
- If serving with the rice, easy cook the rice according to the packet instructions.
- Mix together the olives, pine nuts and red pepper.
- Once the rice is easy cook ed, stir through the olive mix.
- Pile the salsa verde on top of the salmon fillets. Serve with the rice.

109

Apple And Celeriac Soup

- 2 apple, chopped 4 tablespoons vegetable stock
- 600ml almond or coconut milk
- pepper and salt to taste
- 2 tbsp avocado or olive oil
- 2 onion diced 2 clove of garlic
- 2 leek finely chopped 600g celeriac, peeled and diced

1. In a large pan, heat the oil and sauté the onion, garlic, and leek for two to three minutes.

2. Add in the remaining ingredients.

3. Bring to a boil, then cover and simmer for twenty minutes, or until the celeriac is completely tender.

4. Blend the ingredients with a stick blender and season to taste.

111

5. Add more water or almond milk as required to thin.

Stir-Fried Beef Negmak With Green Beans And Watersre

Ingredients

2 tablespoon clover honey or pure maple syrup

Coconut or avocado oil

16 ounces French green beans, cut in half

2 bunch scallions, green parts only, cut into 2 -inch pieces

10 ounces watercress
2 pound flank steak

Sea salt

½ cup sake or dry white wine (optional)

½ cup gluten-free tamari or coconut aminos

4 tablespoons rice or white wine vinegar

Instructions

1. Slice the steak as thinly as possible against the grain.
2. Season generously with salt. Set aside.

3. In a small bowl, stir together the sake tamari, vinegar, and honey until dissolved.

4. Set a large wok or heavy-bottomed skillet over high heat.

5. Add a thin layer of oil and arrange the steak in an even layer.

6. Brown the meat, flipping once, until there's a dark sear on both sides, about 5-10 minutes total.

7. Transfer to a bowl.

8. Add the green beans and sauce to the pan. Simmer vigorously, stirring occasionally, until the sauce has reduced by half and the beans are al dente, about 5-10 minutes.

9. Return the beef to the pan along with the scallions and toss to coat in the sauce.

10. To serve, arrange the watercress on a platter and top with the beef stir-fry and sauce.

11. Serve immediately alongside white rice, if you like.

Fodu's Low FODMAP Veggie Fried Rise with Teriuaki Sause

Ingredients:

2 cup snow peas

2 whole red pepper, diced

1 cup pineapple chunks

2 tablespoon ground ginger

½ cup

8 cups cooked white rice 4 cups shredded carrots

1 cup scallions greens

Fody's Low FODMAP Teriyaki Sauce

Fody's Shallot-Infused Olive Oil

6 large eggs, beaten Sesame seeds + scallion greens for garnish

½ cup soy sauce

2 tbsp sesame oil

4 tbsp

Directions

1. Pre-heat oven to 450 F and thoroughly grease a baking sheet.
2. In a large mixing bowl, toss together rice and your Low FODMAP vegetables.
3. In a small mixing bowl, whisk ground ginger, Fody Teriyaki Sauce, soy sauce, sesame oil, and Fody Shallot-Infused Olive Oil until combined.
4. Drizzle dressing over rice and vegetable mixture, continuing to mix + toss until rice and veggies are fully coated.
5. Evenly spread the rice mixture on the baking sheet and bake for 25-30 minutes until the rice begins to toast.
6. Once rice is beginning to toast, using a spatula, toss the rice on the pan, turning to ensure it evenly cooks.
7. Drizzle beaten fresh eggs over top of rice mixture and continue baking an

additional 25 to 30 minutes until the fresh eggs are cooked.

8. Garnish with sesame seeds and scallion greens before serving.

9. Voila, your Low FODMAP vegetable fried rice is all set!

www.ingramcontent.com/pod-product-compliance
Lightning Source LLC
Chambersburg PA
CBHW060517030426
42337CB00015B/1924